EVERY MAN
OUR NEIGHBOR

EVERY MAN OUR NEIGHBOR

A Brief History of the
Massachusetts General Hospital

1811-1961

by

JOSEPH E. GARLAND

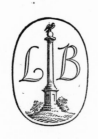

LITTLE, BROWN AND COMPANY

Boston   *Toronto*

Published simultaneously in Canada
by Little, Brown & Company (Canada) Limited

PRINTED IN THE UNITED STATES OF AMERICA

Foreword

The one hundred and fiftieth birthday of the eldest daughter of the Harvard Medical School is a double celebration. For it has always seemed to me that the founding of the Massachusetts General Hospital marked the passing of Harvard from its youth as a small provincial college to the greater maturity of a university.

Every useful institution develops in response to a social need. Harvard Medicine was born on the battlefields of the American Revolution. "The groans of the sick and wounded, suffering and perhaps dying for want of necessities," echoed in the ears of Dr. John Warren, Surgeon of the Continental Army, and within a decade he responded eagerly to the call from Harvard College to help organize a Medical School. He became in 1782 the first Professor of Anatomy and Surgery.

Had those early Harvard professors — John Warren, Benjamin Waterhouse, Aaron Dexter, John Collins Warren and James Jackson — been content to teach in the cradle of the Yard, there could have been no Harvard Medicine. It was soon vividly clear to them that — if doctors were to have adequate educational opportunities in New England — if their community was to have adequate medical care — there would have to be a hospital. Without the Massachusetts General Hospital, and the constellation of teaching hospitals that has since grown up, the Harvard Medical School would be about as effective as the bridge at Avignon — or one half of the Longfellow Bridge.

Good medicine, great medicine — the tradition of great medicine in Massachusetts is virtually as old as the nation — is rather like the nail for want of which the shoe was lost. Without patients to care for, there is no medicine. Without research, there is no new knowledge with which to improve the care of patients. Without education, there are no new doctors to care for the patients and to push forward in the endless search for knowledge.

Thus, we are always coming full-circle as we try to describe the interdependence of medical school and teaching hospital, wherein resides the effectiveness of the university medical school and the associated, although independent, teaching hospital. The history of the Massachusetts General Hospital and the Harvard Medical School is one of continuous interaction; each has nourished the other for a century and a half.

The late Alan Gregg, one of the wisest of medical statesmen, often compared this relationship to the human arm, whose usefulness is derived from its joints, its lack of rigidity.

Although geography can never be completely overcome, it has long since ceased to exert any major influence on the mutual development of the MGH and the Medical School. The personality of the Hospital — distinctive and strong as an organic part of the community and of the medical profession — will continue to provide, as it always has, a great share of the vigor and achievement of Harvard Medicine. Certainly this partnership has given Boston the "medical consciousness" that in turn has helped to produce our sister medical schools at Boston and Tufts Universities and their teaching hospitals. As Harvard and the MGH move toward a second centennial, the interdependence of their partnership — the articulation of Alan Gregg's "arm" — is daily more significant and imperative.

The Massachusetts General is one of the world's great hospitals, one of the finest achievements of American medicine, a torch of hope for suffering humanity. Something of the meaning of this wonderful place and the sweep of its history emerge from the short book that follows.

Increasing demands are being made on American medicine — strident calls for more doctors, for better health in the years ahead for all people, for faster progress in the fight against disease. None of these demands can be satisfied, however, without the best of medical education, resting securely on the basic sciences and on the actual experience of learning in the atmosphere of a great teaching hospital. For it is in the wards and clinics, the sick rooms and operating theaters, that the medical student becomes a doctor.

A nineteenth century "alumnus" of the MGH once described his "Alma Mater" as a place where the constant search after truth was entirely unsullied by the passions and prejudices of men. As the medical students and young doctors in training today and tomorrow can continue to view their experiences there with the same feeling of admiration and attachment of their predecessors, they will participate in medical education at its best. The best in medical education and the most devoted allegiance to humanity have been the measure of the Massachusetts General Hospital for one hundred and fifty years.

George Packer Berry, M.D.
Dean of the Faculty of Medicine
Harvard University

January 6, 1961

Preface

About four months ago it occurred to some of the people who were planning the 150th Anniversary of the Massachusetts General Hospital that a short, more or less readable story of its history did not exist. Four consecutive accounts — adding up to two thousand pages (and the mountain from which most of the molehill that follows was sifted) — had been capably written, but they do not constitute in the aggregate an easy evening's entertainment or instruction. A bird's eye view was needed, and I agreed to be the bird. The result is a kind of a sketch; it touches on the high points and avoids detail, and is intentionally inferential rather than comprehensive.

Not so long ago one of the elder statesmen on the staff noticed as he was traversing the service area behind the Bulfinch Building a battered old Victorian desk amongst a heap of castoffs being readied for the dump. He rescued it in a nick and had it removed to the Archives Room. For scores of years this had been the House Pupils' desk, and by tradition they had scratched their names on the under side of the wooden lift-top. The signatures of generations of aspiring young doctors were there, men who were to distinguish themselves in American medicine. And it had been junked.

The incident is suggestive of the elusively unique side of the MGH. It is downright absent-minded about its past because it is immersed in the present.

My great-grandfather, while a medical student in 1848, attended teaching clinics at the Massachusetts General Hospital. My grandfather was a House Pupil there, and my father met my mother while he was a House Officer and she a Nurse. Thus I

ix

feel that I am genetically a hybrid of the MGH, although I am
not a doctor. My authorship will have been justified if it adds to
the reader's understanding of the place the Massachusetts
General Hospital occupies in our society.

I am indebted for their suggestions in the preparation of this
manuscript to Doctors Edward D. Churchill, Dean A. Clark,
Joseph Garland and James Howard Means; to David C. Crockett
and Francis W. Hatch; and to R.C.G., my best editor.

J.E.G.

Gloucester, Massachusetts
January 1961

When in distress, every man becomes our neighbor . . .

From a circular letter by Doctors
James Jackson and John Collins
Warren urging the establishment
of a general hospital in Boston.
August 20, 1810.

Contents

CHAPTER 1

Birth of a Heritage

A City Without a Hospital

A hundred and sixty years ago, when the Republic was yet an infant and Boston had but 25,000 inhabitants, the hardiness of the pioneer and a measure of luck were the best insurance of a long life. The average citizen counted himself fortunate if he could avoid the services of the doctor, whose treatment was likely to be worse than the disease. There was no hospital in New England for the general public, and this was just as well, for hospitals in those days were one step removed from the grave-yard.

Most people, when they fell sick, took to their beds and home remedies. If these failed, and a doctor was called, he would solemnly prescribe the therapy of the day — bleeding, purging and puking — an abomination that as a rule succeeded in sabotaging whatever defenses against disease the patient had left.

In 1800 there were only two general hospitals in the young nation, the Pennsylvania Hospital, which Benjamin Franklin helped to found in Philadelphia and which opened in 1756, and the New York Hospital, which opened in 1791. Otherwise, "hospitals" were points of last resort and no return, expedient facilities for the herding-together of smallpox victims during the periodic epidemics that swept the colonies, or assembly areas for what little treatment and solace could be given the sick and

1

wounded Revolutionary soldiers. A marine hospital was to be established in Charlestown in 1804, but it was open only to sailors.

The Boston Dispensary had been started in 1796 for the ambulatory treatment of the poor, but the plain fact is that there was no facility in all of New England where anyone, rich or poor, could receive constant, supervised medical care. The only recourse in the case of the poor of Boston was to carry them to the Almshouse, a desperate and dreaded prospect. For here were thrown together, under incredibly crowded and filthy conditions, the paupers, the indigent sick and the mentally ill of the city.

REVEREND BARTLETT CALLS A MEETING

This, then, was the unhappy picture of medicine in Boston, and indeed, in all of the New World, at the beginning of the nineteenth century, and it preyed on the compassionate mind of the Reverend John Bartlett, Chaplain of the Almshouse, as he met misery, anguish and hopelessness at every turn in his efforts to bring some small comfort to the inmates.

After visiting the hospitals in New York and Philadelphia, and studying new ideas that were coming out of Europe about the treatment of the mentally ill, Reverend Bartlett called a meeting of prominent and powerful Bostonians on March 8, 1810, and urged fervently that they organize a general hospital for the care of the physically and mentally ill.

Years later Reverend Bartlett wrote his son that he had been especially concerned about the treatment of the insane in the Almshouse:

> A 20-foot building, with several cells opening into a long entry, in each of which cells was a board cabin or berth, with loose straw, a pail for necessary purposes, was their only accommodation. The violent were confined in strait jackets, and the filth and wretchedness of the place were dreadful.

It happened that the time was ripe. Among those at the Reverend Bartlett's meeting were two of the town's leading young doctors who had been worrying about the same problem and who needed, apparently, only the inspiration of the chaplain to turn their ideas to action.

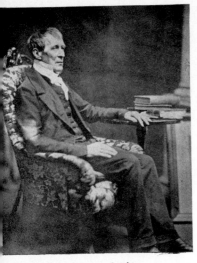

Dr. James Jackson

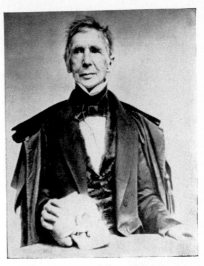

Dr. John Collins Warren

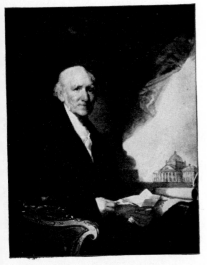

Lt. Gov. William Phillips
(Portrait by Gilbert Stuart)

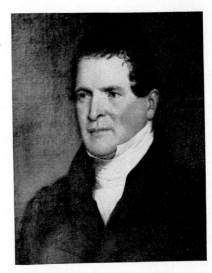

Reverend John Bartlett

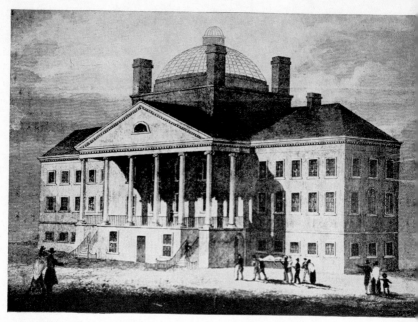

An old print of the Bulfinch Building

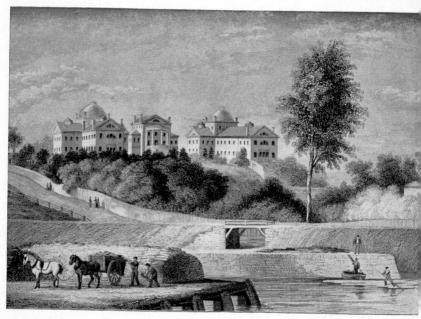

The original McLean Hospital in Somerville

One was Dr. James Jackson, son of a Newburyport merchant, student of the intrepid old Dr. Edward Augustus Holyoke of Salem and a rising, progressive physician and teacher who was to practice in Boston for another half-century.

Kind, tactful and dignified, Dr. Jackson in his dress and habits was the epitome of a gentleman of the old school. He was so punctual in meeting engagements that he always carried two watches. Yet he was a medical freethinker, an innovator, a scientist and clinician of fertile imagination and insight, influential and beloved in and outside his profession. Dr. Oliver Wendell Holmes wrote of Dr. Jackson that he considered it his duty "to stand guard at every avenue that disease might enter, to leave nothing to chance; not merely to throw a few pills and powders into one pan of the scales of Fate, while Death the skeleton was seated in the other, but to lean with his whole weight on the side of life, and shift the balance in its favor if it lay in human power to do it."

Dr. John Collins Warren had been Dr. Jackson's junior by one year at Harvard College and was the second Professor of Anatomy and Surgery at Harvard Medical School (then known as the Massachusetts Medical College). He had succeeded his father, Dr. John Warren, who was the first to hold this chair when the School was founded in 1782. The elder Dr. Warren, first in a distinguished line of Warrens who were to serve the Massachusetts General Hospital and Harvard Medical School for generations, was the brother of the dashing patriot and Revolutionary War hero, Dr. Joseph Warren, who was killed in the Battle of Bunker Hill.

Dr. Warren, like Dr. Jackson, had studied extensively in Europe and throughout his long career maintained close communication with progress in surgery abroad. Ambitious, hardworking and aggressive, he rose to be one of the foremost surgeons in America while still a young man. He was entirely matter of fact in his attitude toward his work and life. At the age of 68, after performing publicly for the first time in the world a surgical operation using ether anesthesia, he turned to his colleagues in the amphitheatre of the Massachusetts General Hospital and declared: "Gentlemen, this is no humbug." Dr. Warren was especially adept at the treatment of fractures, dislocations and aneurysms. He once amputated the lower leg of a patient in forty seconds, the only relief from pain (this was before ether) being pressure on the femoral nerve. He wrote the first American treatise on tumors. With Dr. Jackson he founded in 1812 the *New England Journal of Medicine and Surgery* (now the world-famous *New England Journal of Medicine*), established the Warren Anatomical Museum at Harvard Medical School, was several times president of the Massachusetts Medical Society and the third president of the American Medical Association, which he helped to found.

THE CORNERSTONE OF THE HOSPITAL

As the result of Reverend Bartlett's meeting, Doctors Jackson and Warren were appointed to take the initiative in seeking broad financial support from the wealthy of Boston for the establishment of a hospital. Accordingly, on August 20, 1810, they jointly addressed a circular letter to rich and influential citizens suggesting that the necessary funds could be raised immediately "if a few opulent men will contribute only their superfluous income for one year."

The young doctors had thought their plan out carefully and knew exactly what they wanted. For one thing, they were well aware of the progress that was being made in the improvement of European hospitals, especially in France and England, and they foresaw the advantages that an up-to-date hospital would have in making available proper medical care for their fellow citizens.

Fully as important in their eyes, however, and perhaps even more so in the long run, was the effect that the opening of a hospital in Boston would have in raising the standards of medical education in New England and thus insuring a steady growth in the number of the region's well trained practitioners.

Hence, after presenting several cogent reasons why a hospital was essential to the welfare of the community, Doctors Jackson and Warren noted:

The means of medical education in New England are at present very limited, and totally inadequate to so important a purpose. . . . Those who are educated in New England have so few opportunities of attending to the practice of physic, that they find it impossible to learn some of the most important elements of the science of medicine, until after they have undertaken for themselves the care of the health and lives of their fellow-citizens. This care they undertake with very little knowledge, except that acquired from books . . . With such deficiencies in medical education, it is needless to show to what evils the community is exposed. . . . A hospital is an institution absolutely essential to a medical school, and one which would afford relief and comfort to thousands of the sick and miserable. On what other objects can the superfluities of the rich be so well bestowed?

The response to this letter, which has been called the cornerstone of the Hospital, was immediate and enthusiastic. Within six months — on February 25, 1811 — the Massachusetts Legislature (or General Court, as it is still called) granted a charter for the incorporation of the Massachusetts General Hospital to James Bowdoin and fifty-five other prominent Bostonians. The first meeting of the Corporation was held on April 23, with ex-President of the United States John Adams as moderator.

A WISE (AND GENEROUS) LEGISLATURE

The report of the legislative committee which recommended approval of the charter embodied the objectives set forth in the Jackson-Warren letter and commented that "it is the duty of enlightened Legislators, to provide not only for the present generation, but to be active and vigilant in advancing the happiness of their posterity." It reveals that the purposes for which the Massachusetts General Hospital was established have remained essentially unchanged for 150 years.

The Hospital, thus established, is intended to be a receptacle for patients from all parts of the Commonwealth, afflicted with diseases of a peculiar nature, requiring the most skilful treatment, and presenting cases for instruction in the study and practice of surgery and physic. Among the unfortunate objects of this charitable project, particular provision is to be made for such as the wisdom of Providence may have seen fit to visit with the most terrible of all human maladies — a deprivation of reason. . . .

Persons of every age and sex, whether permanent residents of the town, or occasional residents therein, citizens of every part of the Commonwealth, as well as strangers, from other states and countries, those in indigent circumstances, who, while in health, can gain by their labour a subsistence for themselves and their families, but, when assailed by disease are deprived of the ordinary comforts of life . . . these are among that wretched portion of the community, for whom it is intended to open a tranquil and comfortable asylum. . . .

But it is not to the indigent alone that the advantages of this institution are to be extended. Experience in other states has proved that persons requiring the best surgical and medical aid and having the means of defraying the moderate expenses incident to such a situation will frequently, from choice, resort to a Hospital, as furnishing the most convenient accommodations, and the surest means of restoration to health. . . .

When it is considered how great a portion of the population of the town of Boston is composed of mechanics, journeymen and apprentices, labourers, and domestic servants, mere sojourners in the city with no connections near at hand ready to pour oil and wine into their wounds when they are in need of relief, it cannot be doubted that the plan of a general hospital is the offspring of a liberal and expansive benevolence, ranging far beyond the confines of a single town, and seeking for objects of solace and comfort among the whole family of man! . . .

The location of the proposed Hospital is intended to be such as will accommodate students in the metropolis and at the University in Cambridge, and the skill thus acquired, by the increased means of instruction, will be gradually and constantly diffused through every section of the Commonwealth.

These passages from this historic report are worth studying. They are significant. They define the purpose of our modern voluntary hospital system. They spell out a bill of rights for the sick in a free society. They show that the Massachusetts General Hospital was established for the benefit of all worthy persons, regardless of their citizenship or station in life or economic means, that it was meant to be a *general* hospital in respect to its availability to the *general* population, that its doors were to be opened to "the whole family of man," not merely to the citizens of Boston or Massachusetts.

It augured well for the Hospital that many of its founders were highly influential in the state government; the Legislature proceeded to grant the Corporation rather extraordinary privileges, insisting only that the governor retain the right to appoint four of the twelve trustees and that the Hospital agree to care for thirty physically and mentally ill patients at state expense, a condition that was repealed later.

First the Legislature presented the Hospital with the Province House with the option of disposing of this estate and using the proceeds on the condition that it raise $100,000 by private subscription within five years. The Province House was built in 1679 near the Old South Meeting House by Peter Sargeant and sold in 1716 to the Provincial Legislature, which used it until the Revolution as the residence of the Provincial Governors. Later the State maintained it as a Government House until it was given to the Hospital. In 1817 the Hospital leased it to David Greenough for ninety-nine years for a lump sum of $33,000, and when it reverted to the Hospital in 1916 the value of the property was estimated at more than $1,500,000.

Then, in 1814, the Legislature took a most unusual step. It gave the Corporation of the Hospital the right to go into the life insurance business as a source of additional income. Four years later the Massachusetts Hospital Life Insurance Company was chartered with the provision that one-third of its net profits be turned over to the Hospital. Although these arrangements subsequently took a more conservative turn, they provided the Hospital during the course of the next 130 years with more than $1,500,000 in income. Incidentally, the Massachusetts Hospital Life Insurance Company, founded primarily as a fund-raising device, soon extended its activities into investment and banking, came to have a powerful influence on the industrial development of New England and has taken its place in history as the earliest forerunner of both the modern trust and investment companies.

As if this were not enough, the Legislature continued to bestow favors on the Hospital, including a directive that the State Prison furnish the stone for its first building (worth about $30,000) and an order exempting the superintendent and medical staff from military service.

The injuries inflicted on Boston's commerce by the War of 1812 delayed plans for raising funds to meet the Legislature's Province House condition, but finally, in December 1816, a public fund campaign was launched. Donations were received from citizens in all walks of life, and by March of the following year more than $107,000 had been received from 1047 contributors. The smallest was recorded as 25 cents, the largest as $20,000 from Lt. Gov. William Phillips, a gift that included a $5000 bequest in 1801 from his father, also William Phillips, to be used by the town for the erection of a hospital.

Two of the most bizarre gifts to the Massachusetts General Hospital during its early years were a sow "of an uncommonly fine breed" whose weight was recorded by the Trustees as 273 pounds, and, of all things, a mummy from Thebes. The mummy was a sensation. The ingenious Trustees leased it out for exhibition and netted $1200; its three donors were gratefully elected to the Corporation, and the mummy has remained on display ever since.

OPENING OF THE McLEAN HOSPITAL

The founders and early supporters of the Massachusetts General Hospital were at least as concerned with the mentally ill as they were with the physically sick. In fact, the Trustees assigned priority to the opening of an insane asylum and in 1816 purchased the 18-acre Joy, or Barrell, estate in Charlestown (later to become part of Somerville), consisting of a colonial house designed by Charles Bulfinch atop a lovely hill overlooking Miller's River, a small tributary of the Charles River. The mansion was altered and enlarged for an administration house. Two adjoining buildings were erected, with a capacity of sixty patients.

Dr. Rufus Wyman, a country doctor with a local reputation for handling the mentally ill, was chosen the first superintendent in March 1818, and on October 6 the first patient was admitted — "a young man whose father thought him possessed of the devil, which he had tried to exorcise with the rod." Subsequently he was discharged cured, became a peddler and acquired a small fortune.

A hospital devoted exclusively to the treatment of the mentally ill was a novelty and regarded with some suspicion by the public. It represented a sharp break with the past marked since time immemorial by the brutality and inhumanity which is the inevitable outcome of ignorance and superstition. The asylum, later known as the McLean Hospital, was one of the very first institutions in America to concentrate on the treatment rather than the custodial care of the mentally ill.

Dr. Wyman, and after his retirement Dr. Luther V. Bell, left a lasting mark on the early development of the asylum, whose financial success was assured by John McLean, a Boston merchant who left the institution $25,000 in 1823 and eventually a total of nearly $120,000 from his estate. In his honor it was named the McLean Asylum for the Insane in 1826 and rechristened McLean Hospital in 1892.

Dr. Wyman's "system of moral management" of the mentally ill which was followed devotedly by Dr. Bell would be considered progressive even by today's standards. Both men deplored the use of restraint in any form, and kindness toward patients was the strictest rule of the hospital. Great emphasis was placed upon occupational therapy. Productive work, games and diversions and outdoor exercise were made a way of life, all of which, Dr. Wyman reported as early as 1822, "have a powerful effect in tranquilizing the mind, breaking up wrong associations of ideas and inducing correct habits of thinking as well as acting."

THE HOSPITAL IN PRINCE'S PASTURE

Meanwhile, plans for the Massachusetts General Hospital moved forward. Four acres of a field on the bank of the Charles River in the West End of Boston, known as Prince's Pasture, were acquired; and Charles Bulfinch, the leading architect of the period and designer of the State House and many other famous public and private buildings, was chosen to plan the hospital structure. Bulfinch incorporated central heating and plumbing in this classically conceived granite edifice, which is as solid as the day it was completed. The Bulfinch Building remains today a still-used memorial to the past, dwarfed but not overshadowed by the great hospital complex that has risen all around it.

Captain Nathaniel Fletcher, a retired Newburyport ship's master who had amassed a fortune only to lose most of it as a result of the Embargo Act and the War of 1812, was appointed superintendent and his wife matron on April 1, 1821. Doctors Jackson and Warren had already been asked to be Physician and Surgeon in 1817.

The Massachusetts General Hospital admitted its first patient, a 30-year-old sailor, on September 3, 1821. Eighteen more patients were received during the next four months, 122 the following year, and in 1823 the building was completed to its capacity of 73 beds.

By 1830 the quality of the care given the patients at the Massachusetts General Hospital was comparable to that at the Pennsylvania and New York Hospitals, and the MGH and Harvard Medical School were the dominant medical institutions in New England. The personalities of Doctors Jackson and Warren forcefully moulded the developing character of the Hospital until their retirements in 1837 and 1852, and the course upon which they set it has been followed to this day.

Although Dr. Jackson initiated no radical departures from the therapeutic modes of his time, his methods of treatment were relatively mild and conservative, and there was considerably less emphasis on bleeding, purging and puking than in the country-side generally.

This and other rather terrible medical holdovers from the Middle Ages were finally knocked into limbo in 1835 when Dr. Jacob Bigelow, a physician at the MGH for many years and one of the most brilliant scientific intellects in America, published his classic "A Discourse on Self-Limited Diseases." Dr. O. W. Holmes later wrote that this "did more than any other work or essay in our own language to rescue the practice of medicine from the slavery of the drugging system which was a part of the inheritance of the profession."

Doctors Jackson and Warren vigorously advocated using the

Hospital for clinical research, and Dr. Jackson carried on a number of investigations at the bedside, especially of typhoid fever. The idea that research could and should be undertaken in a hospital was novel at that time, and the MGH was one of the few in the world where it was implemented in a planned way.

As soon as the Massachusetts General Hospital opened its doors in 1821, students from the Harvard Medical School followed their professors from the Boston Almshouse, where they had received clinical instruction under the worst possible conditions, to the wards of the Hospital where they could observe the lessons of their texts put into effect under the best circumstances obtainable in New England.

By the end of its first active quarter century, the Massachusetts General Hospital and its division for the care of the mentally ill had fulfilled the immediate goals of the founders and the Legislature. It was providing as good care for the sick of Boston and New England as could be found in America. As the training ground for the students of Harvard College's medical school it had established Boston as an independent center of medical education on a par with New York and Philadelphia.

CHAPTER 2

Anesthesia, Asepsis and Appendicitis

WATERS OF FORGETFULNESS

If the year 1846 was decisive in the expansion of the American republic, it was nearly as climactic for the newly awakened interest in science out of which an original and independent tradition of achievement was being created in the United States. In this year, at the Massachusetts General Hospital, occurred one of the greatest events in the history of medicine and the first important, entirely American contribution to medical science.

This was the first public demonstration that a chemical agent, sulphuric ether, could be used to eradicate the pain of a surgical operation. Since time immemorial agony and physical shock had been the cost of surgery. Now it was all over. Henceforth the patient would sleep, his body calm and relaxed, leaving the surgeon free to apply his skill to the utmost.

On October 16, 1846, Dr. John C. Warren in the operating theatre of the Bulfinch Building removed a tumor from under the jaw of Gilbert Abbott, who slept under ether and who declared upon awakening that he had felt no pain during the operation. The amphitheatre was crowded with dumbfounded doctors and medical students. The announcement of the efficacy of anesthesia (a word coined later by Dr. Oliver Wendell Holmes) brought worldwide fame to this small hospital, barely thirty-five years old.*

*It is unfortunate that this blessing to humanity was attended by a tragic controversy over who should receive credit for the discovery.

Dr. Crawford W. Long, a Georgia general practitioner, had used ether in a few minor operations in 1841 but became discouraged and failed to publish his results.

13

⌊ "The fierce extremity of suffering has been steeped in the waters of forgetfulness," wrote Dr. Holmes of ether anesthesia, "and the deepest furrow in the knotted brow of agony has been smoothed forever." ⌋

A single brutal example, recounted by Nathaniel I. Bowditch in his early history of the Hospital, will suffice to suggest the meaning of this event for humanity:

> But a few years ago, and on one occasion of almost every week at the Hospital, deep groans of distress or sharp cries of agony penetrated into the innermost recesses of the building, and were often distinctly audible through the neighborhood. Now, the performance of the severest and gravest duties of the surgeon awakens only the faint murmur of a dreamy unconsciousness.
>
> I will mention but one instance, perhaps as striking as the lapse of coming years can ever produce. A young lady was admitted with a tumor extending from the upper to the under surface of the tongue, which it had become necessary to extirpate. Dr. Hayward administered ether. A steel hook was then inserted into the tongue, to prevent its being withdrawn by an involuntary muscular movement. Next the tumor was cut out. To stop the effusion of blood, a red-hot iron was then passed three successive times into the cavity, which was finally filled with a piece of sponge. The patient was then asked how she felt; and her reply was, "Very comfortable." She had known nothing of all that had been done. What would otherwise have been torture indescribable had been by her unfelt. In a few days she was well enough to leave us.

The demonstration at the Massachusetts General Hospital that ether could produce complete insensibility to pain was the first of three milestones in the development of modern surgery. The

---

Dr. Horace Wells, a Hartford, Connecticut, dentist, after administering nitrous oxide successfully during tooth extractions, was permitted by Dr. Warren to demonstrate it before his Harvard Medical School class in 1844 but failed to produce complete insensibility and was laughed out of Boston.

It was another dentist, Dr. William T. G. Morton, who gave ether to Gilbert Abbott with his own apparatus and to whom history accords credit for the courage and imagination to demonstrate the chemical's properties in public. Dr. Morton first learned of these characteristics while staying at the Boston home of Dr. Charles T. Jackson, an eminent, eccentric and irascible chemist. After the event Dr. Jackson bitterly assailed Dr. Morton and pressed his claims for credit all the way to Congress and President Franklin Pierce. Morton died a hounded and tragic figure. Jackson lost his mind. Long was ruined in the Civil War and died in disillusion. And Wells, the addicted victim of his experiments with chloroform, committed suicide in a New York prison following a street brawl.

second was the contribution of antiseptic surgery by Joseph Lister of Scotland, inspired by Louis Pasteur's germ theory of disease and popularized in America at the MGH. The third was the discovery by Dr. Reginald H. Fitz of the Massachusetts General Hospital of the true nature of appendicitis and his conclusion that the patient's life can be saved by a radical operation; this paved the way for a new field of surgery in which appendectomy was but the opening wedge.

CLEAN SURGERY COMES TO AMERICA

The abolition of pain was necessary but not sufficient for progress in surgery. The fifth-columnist that might bring all of the surgeon's skill to naught — infection — still stalked the hospital wards.

If the operation was a success, why did so many patients die? For all their art, the surgeons of the mid-nineteenth century remained at a loss to understand the source of the ghastly infections which seemed to appear from nowhere in even the smallest surgical wounds of patients after the most deft operations of which the greatest men of the day were capable. The wound would fester, the infection would spread, and the patient who one day was recovering so well the next day was dying in agony, or if he was lucky, left with weeks of agonizing convalescence.

A description of the preparations for surgery at the MGH before the introduction of antisepsis by Lister has been left us by Dr. J. Collins Warren, the eminent grandson of Dr. John C. Warren; and they were typical of the best hospitals of the period:

> So far as the field of operation was concerned, no preparation of a patient for operation was thought necessary. An examination would be made of the patient's general condition and attention paid to the digestive apparatus. The importance of an "ether breakfast" was recognized. The instruments were kept in plush-covered cases and it was the province of the house pupil to wash them himself after the operation and replace them. It was his duty also to attend to the "layout" for an operation. This consisted, in addition to the requisite instruments, in towels fresh from the laundry, compresses of cotton cloth, and bandages. There was also a wooden tray which contained a number of small round sea sponges which had been washed after previous use by one of

the ward tenders and were supposed to be as clean as soap and water could make them. No attempt was made on the part of the operator or his assistants to attain any special personal cleanliness. The surgeon's toilet was regarded as a postoperative ceremony. An old broadcloth frock coat, as I have said, which had seen too much service to be useful for any other purpose was dedicated in future to surgery.

Infection would usually set in after the operation, Dr. Warren wrote. The surgeon would reluctantly remove the stitches and apply a flaxseed poultice. "Laudable pus" would flow freely, and the wound would be considered as doing well if one of the more virulent infections failed to make an appearance. Eventually it would heal — in about six weeks.

This was cross-infection; "hospitalism" it was called, a word that hints at the dread in which hospital surgery was held. Doctors, nurses and personnel — and everything they touched — carried infection from patient to patient, from ward to ward, from operating table to hospital bed and back.

The surgeons at the Massachusetts General Hospital suspected that there was some connection between infection and filth, and they did indeed attempt cleanliness as far as it was apparent to the eye. The Hospital was undoubtedly one of the "cleanest" in existence.

And still the staff and administration of the MGH, as in every other hospital, were driven almost to distraction by the problem of infection. In 1827, for instance, erysipelas, a streptococcus infection, had become so entrenched in the Hospital that all of the patients were moved to the nearby home of a minister while the building was subjected to thorough fumigation.

Periodically over the years successive waves of infection swept through the Hospital. These were thought to be due to poor ventilation and to the stagnation of "putrid human exhalations." Much attention was given to the proper airing of the buildings, and in 1854 a separate structure was erected as an isolation ward for cases "of a foul and dangerous nature." As late as 1862, when the city was filling in the flats of the Charles River at the edge of the Hospital property the odor was regarded —no one seemed to know just why — as a source of infection.

After the discovery of anesthesia, the number of operations increased, but there was no corresponding improvement in technique and, as might be expected, infection became an increasing problem. The Civil War (during which the MGH cared for 483 sick and wounded soldiers) placed great demands on the surgeon and presented him with many opportunities for progress, but at every turn his technique was balked by insidious, uncontrollable infection.

Then, in 1864, Joseph Lister, surgeon to the Glasgow Royal Infirmary, heard that a French scientist, Louis Pasteur, had shown that fermentation was due to the action of minute living organisms. Might not germs also account for the pus that accompanied infection in a wound? Lister found that diluted carbolic acid was an effective antiseptic agent, or germ-killer. First he discovered that by cleaning surgical wounds with a carbolic wash and dressing them with carbolized lint and gauze he could prevent the infection that usually resulted in amputation of a limb following its compound fracture. Then he devised a machine that sprayed a fine mist of carbolic acid in the air over the operating table, with spectacular results. This was the dawn of modern surgery.

It happened that in 1869 young Dr. J. Collins Warren, the grandson of the co-founder and the son of Dr. Jonathan Mason Warren (also an eminent surgeon at the MGH who had introduced plastic surgery to America from Europe), was traveling and studying abroad, and he visited Lister in Glasgow. He was so impressed with what he saw and heard that he brought a sample of Lister's carbolized dressings with him to Boston and enthusiastically set about trying to introduce the antiseptic method at the Massachusetts General Hospital.

Dr. Warren was not the first to give antisepsis a try in America, but he was among the most tenacious. The older surgeons at the MGH were skeptical. Many of the early results were equivocal for lack of precise attention to all of the details of Lister's technique. The assiduous cleanliness and the seemingly cumbersome methods necessary to its success were difficult for the old-time surgeons to understand and put up with. Finally, after a decade of trial and error and constant proselytizing by Dr. Warren, Dr Henry Jacob Bigelow, the senior surgeon at the Hospital and probably the foremost in the United States, was convinced and wholeheartedly espoused "Listerism" which a few years earlier he had opposed.

A whole new world opened up for surgery. Now anesthesia truly came into its own. Lister's experiments were taken up by others, and in Germany emerged the principle of asepsis, the prevention of infection by sterilizing instruments and dressings and clothing with heat. As the patient slept, the surgeon could give rein to the advancement of his technique, sure in the knowledge that the danger of infection had been minimized.

Dr. Fitz Gives the Final Push

Just as asepsis was beginning to catch on in the world of medicine, a man who himself was not a surgeon wrote a paper that gave surgery the final push it needed to emerge as a modern science. Dr. Reginald H. Fitz, the Pathologist and later a Visiting Physician at the Massachusetts General Hospital, published in 1886 a treatise entitled "Perforating Inflammation of the Vermiform Appendix: With Special Reference to Its Early Diagnosis and Treatment." His conclusions were based on an examination of the organs of patients who had died of a mysterious infection that swept through their abdominal cavities and went by a variety of names.

Dr. Fitz proved that this deadly infection originated in the appendix, a vestigial part of the intestine. He called it "appendicitis." He showed that when the swollen and infected appendix bursts it spills bacteria into the abdominal cavity containing the intestine and causes peritonitis, which is often fatal. The way to prevent peritonitis and to cure appendicitis, Dr. Fitz declared, is to remove the appendix by surgery before it has had time to burst.

This historic discovery attained immediate acceptance. Dr. Maurice H. Richardson and other members of the surgical staff of the MGH made early use of an operation for the removal of the appendix — the appendectomy — and led the way in

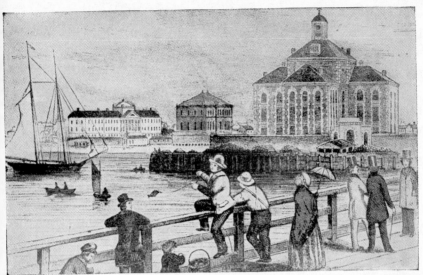

This quaint print shows the Massachusetts General Hospital before the Charles River flats were filled. The Bulfinch Building is at the left, the old Harvard Medical School in center, and the Suffolk County Jail at right. The tower has been removed, but the jail still stands.

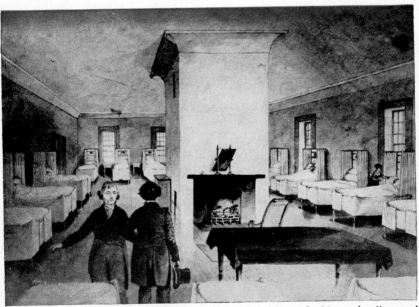

Two frock-coated doctors discuss a case in an old ward. Note the "central heating."

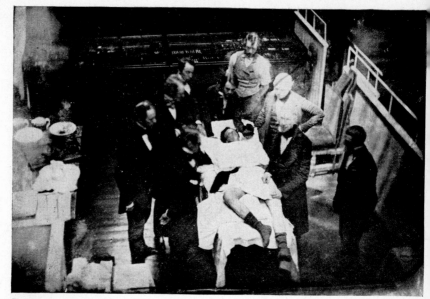

Daguerrotype made a few months after the historic operation in the "Ether Dome" of the Bulfinch Building October 16, 1846. Surgeon with hands resting on the patient's leg is probably Dr. John Collins Warren.

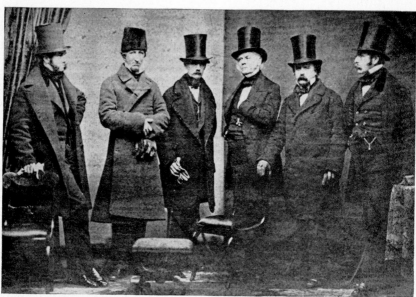

A group of visiting surgeons in 1855. Doctors Henry J. Bigelow, Samuel Cabot, J. Mason Warren, Solomon D. Townsend, George H. Gay and H. G. Clark.

showing their colleagues how to perform it and in demonstrating its effectiveness.

But Dr. Fitz's paper had even wider implications. Because of the great danger of infection involved in any incision of the large area of the abdominal cavity, most surgeons hesitated even to make the attempt. Dr. Fitz forced them to it; if appendicitis was to be cured, an immediate decision as to the necessity of surgery had to be made. Fortunately, his paper appeared hot on the heels of antisepsis and asepsis and pointed the way toward prompt surgical treatment of acute abdominal emergencies.

These were days of ferment and activity at the Massachusetts General Hospital. Three years after Dr. Fitz's paper appeared, a special building, the Bradlee Ward, designed for the performance of abdominal and brain surgery, was opened at the Hospital. It was among the first, if not the first, exclusively aseptic operating facilities in the United States. Appropriately, Dr. J. Collins Warren performed the first operation.

Nursing Becomes a Profession

When Miss Rebecca Taylor retired in 1860 after thirty-four years as head nurse at the Massachusetts General Hospital, Dr. James Jackson was moved to write a tribute to her. If Becky Taylor was at all typical of the kind of nursing service that was provided the patients during the fifty years before any sort of formal training was available, it must have been characterized by kindness and efficiency. Dr. Jackson said of her:

> All, who have known her, will remember the great modesty of her deportment. She never obtruded herself on the notice of any one, and never claimed any distinction. . . . She was uniformly devoted to the sick in her wards, in the most quiet manner, and most tenderly too; but she never substituted terms of endearment for faithful and punctual attendance. . . .
>
> There is not any comparison to be made between our good nurse and Miss Nightingale. The latter is a lady of education, and in a different rank of life. She sees how important is the office of a nurse. She has studied the duties, I may say the high duties of a nurse for the sick.

She has brought science to her aid. . . . My friend is one of much humbler pretensions. She has been a hired nurse. She sought an employment for her living. Having gained an appointment, she gave herself to her duties. Filled with a sense of duty, she brought all her faculties into exercise, without bustle, and without parade. . . . I think if any unhappy and captious individual in her ward had found fault with her, all the other inmates of it would, at once, have risen up in her defence. . . .

It is a pleasure to bear testimony in favor of one so good. I cannot help hoping that it will be useful to hold up such an example for imitation. And, I will add, that, so far as my influence can go, I wish to point out how high are the duties of a nurse; and how justly they entitle one, who performs them skillfully and faithfully and kindly, to the love and respect of mankind.

By the time Becky Taylor had retired from the MGH doctors throughout the civilized world were beginning to practice medicine on a truly scientific basis. With Lord Lister's monumental innovations in the offing, hospitals were on the verge of becoming places of hope rather than desperation.

But nursing remained an arduous, poorly rewarded domestic occupation that required only rudimentary training. As doctors brought the new techniques of science into the hospital, the elements needed in the care of the patients took on a sophistication that could be acquired only through greater nursing skill and education.

We might expect that the doctors themselves would have taken the initiative in raising the standards of a service on which they were so dependent. But they didn't, and many were actually opposed to the upgrading of this feminine occupation. The fact is that nursing matured into a profession as part of a world-wide struggle of women generally to achieve equal status with men.

Miss Florence Nightingale, who was so highly respected by Dr. Jackson, demonstrated during the Crimean War in 1854 what a woman of education and determination could accomplish against apparently devastating odds and five years later made nursing a profession when she organized the world's first training school for nurses at St. Thomas' Hospital in London. Her crusading spirit set fires around the globe, and during the Civil War Clara

Barton, the Angel of the Battlefield, kindled a similar fervor in America.

By 1873 a determined committee of influential ladies in Boston succeeded in overcoming the strenuous objections of the Trustees and visiting staff of the Massachusetts General Hospital and established the Boston Training School for Nurses. It opened with six pupils, and the Hospital dubiously paid $150 a month for the nursing service it provided. The school was the third in the United States connected with a general hospital. Matters proceeded badly until the next year, when Miss Linda Richards, a graduate of the New England Hospital for Women and Children and the first trained nurse in America, was put in charge.

Two years later, however, these first young trained nurses had so demonstrated their competence that the Trustees permitted them to move their school into the abandoned "Old Brick" that had once been an isolation ward, noting as they did so with an air of cautious optimism that the ladies "with right notions of their duties, will eventually prove a blessing to the sick of all classes in the community." And so it came to pass, although it was not for another twenty years — in 1896 — that the conservative Trustees formally adopted the school as the Hospital's own.

THE McLEAN MOVES

Meanwhile, across the river in Somerville, the ladies of Boston were pressing on with a parallel movement, and their persistence in 1882 resulted in the opening at the McLean Hospital of the first training school for nurses in a hospital for the mentally ill anywhere in the world.

Nevertheless, all was not well at the McLean. Although the enlightened spirit of its early superintendents, Doctors Wyman and Bell, continued to guide their successors, the treatment of patients was made increasingly difficult by the absorption of the once pastoral setting of the hospital into the expanding industrial complex of Boston. As the railroads grew to meet the needs of the city, more and more tracks cut across and around the Mc-

Lean's property. By 1871 the hospital was nearly isolated in the middle of a sprawling freight yard surrounded by industries and tenements, and the Trustees decided the time had come to seek greener pastures. In 1875 a large tract of open land was purchased in the Waverley section of Belmont, and after many vicissitudes and delays the McLean Hospital was moved twenty years later to its present spacious home.

GIANTS OF MEDICINE

The half-century stretching from the demonstration of anesthesia in 1846 to the coming of modern research in 1896 saw the Massachusetts General Hospital transformed into an expanding medical center full of the excitement of the approaching new century and in the process of establishing itself as a national institution.

These were years when the Hospital was still small enough — and the science of medicine young enough to be encompassed by the mind of the individual — that its character and future could be identifiably shaped by a succession of great doctors who were also great teachers and innovators.

There was the giant of them all, Dr. Henry Jacob Bigelow, bearded autocrat of American surgery who resigned in 1886 after forty years on the staff, son of Dr. Jacob Bigelow. He was the first to accurately describe the anatomy of the hip joint in reference to dislocation, inventor of an evacuator to wash out fragments of stones after they had been crushed in the bladder, apostle of anesthesia and in time of asepsis, powerful as a proponent and an opponent to be reckoned with.

There was the whimsical Professor of Anatomy at Harvard Medical School who really preferred to write, Dr. Oliver Wendell Holmes. Author of the classic paper in 1842 which pointed out that doctors themselves were responsible for passing childbirth fever from mother to mother, Dr. Holmes was only briefly on the staff of the MGH, but his sagacity was felt for decades, and he spoke for his and succeeding generations when he wrote:

This Hospital has always inspired the fervid attachment of those holding any relationship to it whatsoever, — whether as citizens, proud of its benevolent services; as pupils, grateful for its teachings; or as medical officers, who have put their own work into its comprehensive fields of usefulness. It has universally fostered a feeling of affection, such as is cherished for an Alma Mater.

There were the Warrens, a medical family as indestructible as the Hospital itself, always vital and productive, fathers and sons.

There were Doctors Samuel Cabot and John Homans, who dared to perform ovariotomies (unsuccessfully until antisepsis came along) — but in rented rooms outside the Hospital lest their patients be exposed to the contaminated operating theatre.

There was Dr. Henry I. Bowditch, son of the astronomer and mathematician, who with Dr. Morrill Wyman was among the first to puncture the chest wall in order to remove fluid from the chest. Dr. Bowditch was the first chairman of the Massachusetts Board of Health, which was the first in the United States.

There was Dr. Walter Channing, quick of temper and wit, usher of anesthesia into obstetrics, brother of William Ellery Channing, the clergyman. When a caller one day asked for Dr. Channing, he replied: "Which one? My brother preaches and I practise."

There was Dr. James C. White, whose son and grandson were to follow him on the staff. He was the first dermatologist in America, a specialty he brought back from study in Vienna to introduce as one of the earliest at the MGH, and the moving spirit on the faculty behind the sweeping reform of education at Harvard Medical School in 1870-71.

During these years the bonds between the Massachusetts General Hospital and Harvard Medical School grew stronger and closer, yet remained informal and flexible. It was assumed that every member of the staff of the Hospital was a teacher, passing on the light of his knowledge and experience to the next generation, and that every practising doctor on the faculty of the Medical School was a humanitarian, contributing to the care of the patients at the Hospital.

In the years ahead, the sick of the world and those who would light their own torches of knowledge were to beat a path to Boston.

CHAPTER 3

The Flowering of Research

PATHOLOGY SETS THE STAGE

Fifty years to the day after the first public demonstration of anesthesia — on October 16, 1896 — the Massachusetts General Hospital, with a fine sense of history, formally opened its Pathology Laboratory. In fact, this was the Hospital's first real laboratory of any kind. It was a small undertaking, but it signified recognition by the Trustees that the promotion of science within its walls is a responsibility of the hospital to its patients of the future.

As early as 1854 a hundred dollars had been appropriated to establish a "pathological cabinet," or museum for the preservation of autopsy material, and a curator was appointed to conduct autopsies. Although the importance of this most ancient form of medical research continued to be recognized, both the MGH and Harvard Medical School realized by the early nineties that the new Johns Hopkins Hospital and Medical School in Baltimore were surpassing them in the study and teaching of pathology and bacteriology. Dr. William T. Councilman was called to Harvard from Johns Hopkins, and it was as a result of his advice that the new laboratory was created and Dr. James Homer Wright, one of his brilliant young pupils, was appointed Pathologist at the MGH.

A driving, original investigator who hid his shy gentleness behind a cloak of fierce irritability, Dr. Wright created an air of scientific excitement at the Hospital and started it on the path of modern medical research. His own contributions were

25

formidable, and he is remembered today chiefly for his discovery of the origin of blood platelets and his methods of staining pathological specimens for microscopic study.

Research at the McLean Hospital received its initial stimulus from the superintendent during this period, Dr. Edward Cowles, a former Union Army surgeon who had picked up some incidental knowledge of psychology. Dr. Cowles was responsible for the appointment of Dr. William Noyes as pathologist in 1888, and the next year a laboratory was started with the aim of combining pathology, anatomy, neurology, physiology, psychology and psychiatry in what was probably the first multidisciplined approach to the study of mental illness.

When Dr. Noyes resigned in 1893 he was succeeded by Dr. August Hoch as pathologist and psychologist. Dr. Hoch placed the clinical work of the laboratory on a firm scientific basis and laid the groundwork for the establishment in 1904 of a true psychological laboratory under Dr. Shepherd I. Franz. In the meantime a chemical laboratory had been opened in 1900 under Dr. Otto Folin, later to be appointed Professor of Biological Chemistry at Harvard Medical School.

Thus within the span of fifteen years one of the earliest attempts in the world to put the study of mental illness on a broad scientific footing was launched at the McLean Hospital.

The Saga of Dr. Dodd

One of the earliest applications in America of Professor Wilhelm Roentgen's discovery of the x-ray was at the Massachusetts General Hospital, and the story of the central figure in this development is a poignant and heroic chapter in the Hospital's history.

When Professor Roentgen announced his discovery in December 1895, Walter J. Dodd was the head pharmacist and photographer at the MGH. Dodd, who had a small laboratory known as the Kingsley Studio, was the self-educated son of an English metalworker; he had a scientific bent and was taking courses in chemistry and pharmacology in his spare time.

Within a matter of days after Roentgen's announcement,

Dodd (for it seemed naturally to fall to the photographer) began efforts to produce an x-ray. His attempts of the first few weeks failed. Then, early in 1896, the first dim picture was taken. It is not clear who actually produced it. One version says that it came from an x-ray tube purchased by Dodd. Dr. Harvey Cushing, the eminent brain surgeon who was a house officer at the time, said years later that he and a colleague produced the first x-ray of a hand using a tube brought back from Roentgen's laboratory by Dr. J. Collins Warren.

Whoever may have actually taken the first radiograph, the credit must go to Dodd and the primitive, ingenious, hand-cranked apparatus he assembled.

Dodd quickly replaced the hand-operated static machine with a coil developed by Professor Hermann Lemp of the General Electric Company and used this, adding his own refinements, to take one of the world's earliest satisfactory chest plates. By 1897 Dr. Reginald H. Fitz was able to show a medical convention a radiograph of the entire body of Dodd's assistant, Joseph Godsoe.

The speed with which the diagnostic value of the x-ray was appreciated by the medical staff is indicated in a statement by the Trustees that during 1897 "not only have most of the broken bones been treated by the light of the x-rays, but bullets and other foreign bodies are constantly located in this way. The operation of oesophagotomy has been done four times for coins and whistles caught in the throat."

An early hint of radiation therapy is found in the story of the man who was referred in 1897 from the out-patient department for x-ray examination. A few days later he reported that the "light" had relieved the pain in his leg. After investigating, Dodd and Dr. Seabury W. Allen rightly concluded that x-rays were capable of relieving pain in certain conditions, probably due to changes they effected in the blood supply.

Dodd's fascination with roentgenology spurred him on to the study of medicine, and in 1907, after receiving his medical degree from the University of Vermont, he was appointed the Hospital's first Roentgenologist.

Important though Dr. Dodd's technical achievements were, his ingenuity and imagination in the application of the x-ray to diagnosis and research were even more significant to the development of roentgenology. All of the Hospital relied from the beginning on his interpretations of radiographs, and his participation was considered essential to research with this new scientific tool. He had a magnetic personality and was beloved by everyone at the MGH.

But within a year of his first enthusiastic contact with x-rays his hands were crippled by agonizing radiation burns, and it was necessary for him to be admitted as a patient for a skin grafting operation. His suffering was intense, but he continued his work relentlessly. Five years later he developed cancer as a result of continuous exposure to radiation in those pioneering days when no one had heard of dosage limits or fully comprehended the lethal effects of x-rays. The few years that remained of his life were filled with agony. He submitted to fifty operations under anesthesia and lost his fingers, bit by bit, even as other parts of his body were increasingly affected.

Although Dr. Dodd was still able to perform exceptional service with the wounded in France during 1915, for which he was decorated by the British government, he returned home and died in 1916 after nearly twenty years of physical agony, a martyr to his own courage and imagination.

CLINICAL RESEARCH GROWS UP

The character of medical research by the beginning of the twentieth century was undergoing great changes. A handful of monumental discoveries in all of the sciences — largely the achievement of individual men working on their own — had paved the way and provided the foundation blocks on which an increasingly intricate structure was to be erected. Much of the medical progress of the previous century had been the result of the empirical observations of practising doctors who had dared to try new things in the course of their primary activity, the treatment of patients. Thus did Dr. John C. Warren risk his professional reputation in order to demonstrate ether anesthesia, the Scotch surgeon Joseph Lister evolve his methods of antisepsis and Dr. Frederick C. Shattuck of the MGH come to advocate in 1897 the treatment of typhoid fever patients with a high calorie diet instead of starvation.

The times called for a new kind of scientist-doctor, someone who combined the practice of medicine with a sound knowledge of science and an instinct for experimentation.

Clinical research as we know it today — a kind of two-way exchange of ideas, information and experience between the laboratory and the patient's bedside — really started at the Massachusetts General Hospital in 1912 with the unprecedented appointment of Dr. David L. Edsall of the Washington University School of Medicine in St. Louis as Chief of one of the two medical services and Jackson Professor of Clinical Medicine at Harvard Medical School.

Dr. Edsall's appointment was unusual because he was the first member of the practising staff in the history of the Hospital to come from outside of Boston, so highly regarded was his clinical and research background.

Dr. Edsall wanted research to become a part of the life of the MGH. He wished to inoculate the doctors on the staff with the contagion of scientific curiosity, to see it spread, to encourage them to bring the problems of their patients to the laboratory and the insights of science to the bedside. He set about finding space, gathering funds, and most important, assembling a group of promising young men whom he sent away to other medical centers for special training in preparation for the task ahead.

Those who formed the nucleus of Dr. Edsall's group were Paul Dudley White, who studied cardiology; J. Howard Means, who began to investigate hemodynamics and respiratory physiology; and George R. Minot, who started the research in the problems of blood that in 1934 won him the Nobel Prize for his discovery of the treatment of pernicious anemia by liver. All three won fame in their fields with the passage of time.

WARD 4: EXPERIMENTS WITH HUMANS

These and other men pursued their special interests, working with patients in the general wards of the Hospital, until it became evident that they needed a special ward of their own where cooperative patients with challenging problems could be observed and treated under the actual conditions of the laboratory. In 1924, just before he left the MGH to take the full-time post of Dean of the Harvard Medical School, Dr. Edsall obtained funds to rebuild and enlarge the east end of the Bulfinch Building. A metabolic research ward of ten beds — Ward 4 it was called for no particular reason — was opened there in 1925 under Dr. Means, who shortly before had been appointed Chief of Medical Services.

Ward 4, now famous in the history of medical research, was first used by Dr. Joseph C. Aub to discover the mechanism of lead poisoning and how to treat it successfully. Many courageous patients since that time have volunteered to submit themselves to the experiments of a succession of investigators. In 1949 Ward 4 was renamed in honor of Edward Mallinckrodt, Jr., of St. Louis because of his many benefactions. The lines of research in Mallinckrodt-Ward 4 have never been directed down specific channels but have been allowed to follow whatever direction seemed fruitful.

Numerous metabolic diseases were explored in Ward 4. Dr. Means studied disorders of the thyroid; Dr. Fuller Albright and his associates investigated hyperparathyroidism and other metabolic diseases of bone; and Dr. Walter Bauer began the work which led to his extensive research into arthritis and other diseases of connective tissue. There were many others, and the fascinating story of this human laboratory and the benefits it has given humanity is told by Dr. Means in his book, *"Ward 4."*

TRIBUTARIES SWELL THE STREAM

The coming of Dr. Edsall to the Massachusetts General Hospital was no isolated event. Other factors were already at work, and they were contributing to the upsurge of creative activity that heralded the second century of the Hospital's history.

Originally, Doctors Jackson and Warren had served continuously as chiefs of medicine and surgery. But in 1835 the

Hospital began the policy of rotating visiting physicians and surgeons as chiefs of their services throughout each year. As the years passed and the operation of the Hospital waxed more complex, it was apparent that this practice — with the continual breaks in continuity it involved — was a source of universal dissatisfaction. Finally, in 1908, the MGH returned to the continuous arrangement on the medical services and in 1911 followed suit with the surgical services. The traditional rotation of physicians visiting the wards, however, continues to this day.

These changes were followed in 1912 by a sweeping reorganization with the creation of the General Executive Committee of the Staff, the medical and surgical executive committees being relegated to subordinate but important positions.

This move was most significant for the progress of research. With its broad powers for the coordination of staff activities, the General Executive Committee adopted the principle of "End Results" which had been championed a decade earlier by Dr. E. A. Codman; it became a matter of policy that the results of surgery should be followed up both for the benefit of the patient and for the sake of what might be learned from the outcome of his case. Furthermore, the General Executive Committee encouraged the initiation of "Special Assignments" by members of the staff — opportunities for the imaginative to commence projects with groups of patients in specialized areas that were of interest to them. Out of these Special Assignments grew clinics which deal with problems ranging from allergy and diabetes to thoracic and thyroid disorders.

An effort in surgical research parallel to Dr. Edsall's in medicine was begun in 1922 by Dr. Edward P. Richardson, who brought together a similar nucleus of young surgical investigators which included Doctors Monroe A. McIver, Edward D. Churchill, Robert R. Linton and James C. White. Laboratories for surgical research were opened in 1930 after the reconstruction, supervised by Dr. Churchill, of the west wing of the Bulfinch Building for that purpose.

With Dr. Richardson's appointment clinical investigation

in medicine and surgery became a joint effort, and the main stream of research at the Massachusetts General Hospital swelled and broadened as it was fed by a growing number of tributaries. Within a few years practically every service had a laboratory somewhere in the Hospital.

THE PROLIFERATION OF RESEARCH

World War II brought antibiotics, new surgical techniques and atomic medicine and gave such a spur to research that by 1947 the Hospital seemed about to burst at the seams. The financing of medical investigation was getting to be big business, and the physical plant was less adequate to the job every day. The Research Council which had been formed in 1938 to bring some element of over-all planning into the picture was clearly outmoded, and it was replaced by the Committee on Research comprised of Trustees and staff members. The new group took on the task of coordinating all research in the Hospital, applications for grants and the distribution of funds. In addition, a Scientific Advisory Committee of outside scientists was organized to assist the Trustees and the Research Committee in evaluating the Hospital's program in the context of scientific endeavor generally and to recommend the allocation of funds; its members included Dr. Karl T. Compton, President of Massachusetts Institute of Technology, and representatives from Washington University, the Rockefeller Institute for Medical Research and Harvard Medical School.

The creation of these two committees was unequivocal recognition, if not the culmination, of a trend which had added a new dimension to the character of the Massachusetts General Hospital without altering its objectives. The spirit of research, sparked by men like Wright and Edsall, had invaded every corner of the institution so pervasively that it had long since become a tradition. Initially carried on incidental to the care of patients, research had been gradually given greater emphasis by a handful of staff members who divided their time between the laboratory and their patients as clinical investigators. As the excitement spread, increasing numbers of doctors found themselves fascinated by the challenges of this dual role, so much so that as medical science attained a status of its own, continued progress demanded the development of a core of men and women who could throw all of their time and energies into the basic investigation of the underlying nature of disease.

BASIC SCIENCE COMES TO THE MGH

A start had been made as early as 1891 with the creation of the Dalton Scholarships designed to provide some modest financial support for young men attracted to clinical research. Dr. Frederick C. Shattuck added impetus in 1910 when he gave Harvard Medical School $25,000 to establish the Walcott Fellowship for a research worker in medicine at the Massachusetts General Hospital.

Finding funds to support scientists who receive no personal income from the practice of medicine was and remains a problem. But slowly a group of full-time scientists was assembled at the Hospital. By the end of World War II medical research had sent pipelines into virtually every other branch of science. Biochemists, biologists, physiologists, pharmacologists, nuclear physicists, organic chemists and radiation engineers were setting up shop at the MGH. A wedding of the biological and physical sciences was taking place, and a new science, biophysics, was emerging with the addition of a new member to the Harvard-MGH partnership, the Massachusetts Institute of Technology across the Charles River in Cambridge.

The position of importance that basic research came to occupy at the Hospital in a rather short time is indicated by the award in 1953 of the Nobel Prize in Physiology and Medicine to Dr. Fritz Lipmann for his discovery of co-enzyme A and its significance in intermediary metabolism. Dr. Lipmann came to the MGH in 1941 as Research Chemist, and this highest of all scientific honors was based on the investigations he carried out while he held this post and later while he was head of the Biochemical Research Laboratory and Harvard Medical School Professor of Biological Chemistry at the Massachusetts General Hospital, to give him his full title.

In 1951 a six-story building devoted exclusively to research was opened, and in 1956 further laboratory space was made available with the dedication of the Warren Building honoring the famous family whose name is synonymous with that of the MGH.

The idea of a coordinated scientific attack on mental illness which was originally conceived by Dr. Edward Cowles during his administration of the McLean Hospital was kept alive during a long interim period when research in the field concentrated mainly on treatment rather than basic causes. A distinguished investigator of the biochemistry of mental illness during this era was Dr. John C. Whitehorn, who rose to be Director of Laboratories and then went on to Johns Hopkins to make further contributions in this difficult field. In 1943 a new era arrived with the appointment of Dr. Cecil K. Drinker of the Harvard School of Public Health as Research Consultant. Under Dr. Drinker's leadership the McLean renewed its preoccupation with the scientific investigation of mental illness and in 1946 established a laboratory devoted to basic research in nervous and mental diseases under Dr. Jordi Folch-Pi. Dr. Folch-Pi and Dr. Alfred Pope directed their efforts to untangling the largely unknown chemistry of the brain, while Dr. Mark D. Altschule, appointed Director of Research in Clinical Physiology in 1947, investigated the larger picture of the chemistry of the whole body in relation to mental illness.

NEW DIRECTIONS IN RESEARCH

The demonstration of ether anesthesia at the Massachusetts General Hospital was not an isolated event in scientific progress or a happy coincidence, dramatic and revolutionary though it may have been. It was the culmination — applied to human beings — of a succession of observations in the field of chemistry about the physiological effects of certain gaseous compounds. Likewise, Roentgen's discovery of x-rays was the result of decades of investigation in physics. Medical scientists did not participate to any significant degree in either of these developments. The forward movement of medicine was following its own lines; chemists and physicists, with the exception of the biochemists,

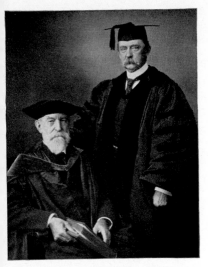

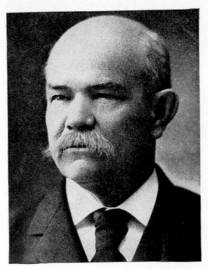

Doctors Henry P. Bowditch
and J. Collins Warren

Dr. Reginald H. Fitz

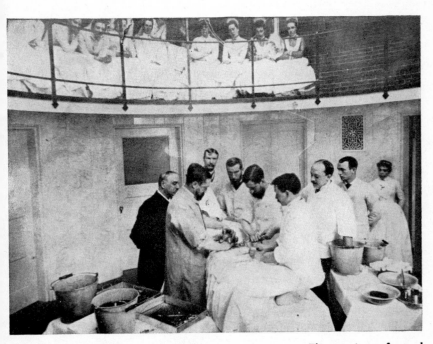

First aseptic operation in the 1889 Bradlee Operating Theater is performed
by Dr. J. Collins Warren, assisted by Dr. Samuel J. Mixter.

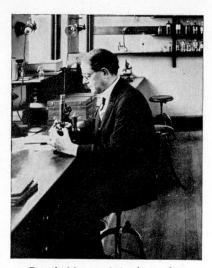
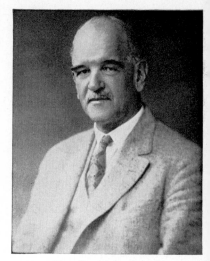

Dr. J. Homer Wright in his
pathology laboratory

Dr. David L. Edsall

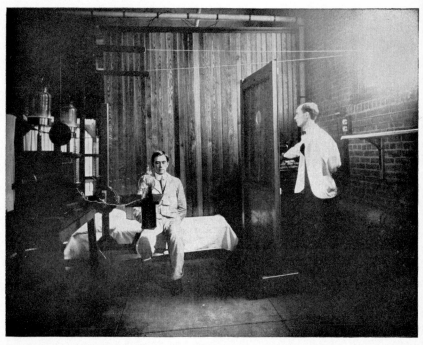

Dr. Walter J. Dodd (right) at the controls of one of his early x-ray machines

were following theirs. Doctors made use of the findings of the non-biological scientists but rarely worked in close concert with them.

But a new approach to medical research had been in the wind for several decades. As early as 1934 the General Executive Committee described what was happening with prophetic insight:

> Professor Cannon (of Harvard Medical School) tells us of the fecundity of aggregation, aggregation of intellects, and President Lowell (of Harvard University) of the stimulating effects of intellectual attrition. In the prosecution of clinical research more and more do we see departmental walls being demolished and men with widely divergent training and interest bringing their minds to focus upon a single problem, uniting their labor to its solution. Such cooperation in research when truly spontaneous, is bound to be fruitful. The association, however, must spring from natural interest and curiosity of the workers. When imposed upon them by someone seeking to compel the investigation of a particular subject, there is apt to be sterility. The quality of research is not strained. It flows from the minds and hands of those who have a special gift for doing it. This its patrons should know so that they may invest in investigators, not in investigation. . . .
>
> In scientific research, perhaps more than in any other field of human endeavor, one thing leads to another. The solving of a problem but opens up a dozen new ones perhaps not even dreamed of before the first was solved. Free choice of problems, and free choice to follow leads disclosed by the solution of a first problem must be the privilege of the researcher. If he strikes a hot scent the means must be found to permit him to follow it with vigor.

If it was becoming clear that the "fecundity of aggregation" depended upon the demolition of walls between clinical investigators at the Hospital, the wisdom of the General Executive Committee applied equally to the more resistant partitions that separated the clinical researchers from the basic scientists, and the biological from the physical sciences. It was apparent that the maintenance of autonomous relationships, wherever they existed, was not producing the new knowledge that medicine required for continued advance.

By 1957 these trends had emerged with sufficient clarity that

Dr. Paul C. Zamecnik, Director of the John Collins Warren Laboratories of the MGH, could express the philosophy of the Committee on Research as follows:

> It was acknowledged that in order to attract and keep basic scientists of high quality, positions of respect and independence would have to be created for them, comparable in nature to those of their clinical colleagues. The field of medical research was thought to be too broad for one pair of legs to span, and it was hoped that a new research idiom would evolve, consisting of a bridge of joined talents. Three types of professional personnel were recognized to be essential to the future of the Hospital as a center for care of patients, teaching, and research: the practitioner busy on the patient front and yet interested in adding to the sum total of knowledge in his special field; the research straddler, engaged in translating the findings of the laboratory into terms of improved human welfare with minimum loss of time; and the Ph.D. and non-clinical M.D. personnel immersed in laboratories but sympathetic to their surroundings.

Still, the fecundity of aggregation. The MGH, which in 1935 had spent $50,000 for research, was financing about 350 different projects in 1960 with more than $4,000,000, a fifth of its total operating budget. They ranged from such clearly practical goals as the development of surgical operations for the correction of heart defects to such fundamental investigations as of the way bone is manufactured by the body.

Yet, as Dr. Nathaniel W. Faxon, Director-Emeritus, wrote in 1959, the line of demarcation between clinical and basic research had disappeared, "and now it is hardly possible to tell where one begins and the other leaves off. Research now is and should be a study without boundaries."

Every brooklet of research at the Massachusetts General Hospital was flowing into a common stream. So was teaching, the passing of knowledge forward to other doctors who would care for other patients, to other scientists who would search out other problems. The stream flowed on without boundaries and without beginning or end.

CHAPTER 4

The Conscience of the Community

A BOSTON HERITAGE

One day about a hundred years ago a little girl was playing on the railroad tracks near the Massachusetts General Hospital when a train roared through and crushed her foot. She was rushed to the Hospital, where it was necessary to amputate her limb.

Trustee Nathaniel I. Bowditch heard of the tragic accident and when she was well enough took the child to a directors' meeting of the railroad, pleaded her case and won a settlement of $300 to be held in trust for her.

Still not content that he had done all he could, Bowditch saw to it that she should live at the Hospital, attend school nearby and eventually be given a lifetime job as a seamstress at the MGH. The child's parents, however, understandably wanted her home, and there she was returned, much to Bowditch's regret.

Perhaps this maimed little girl would have been better off had she been allowed to follow the well-intentioned course that Bowditch had laid out. Her parents were poor immigrants and doubtless were hard put to it to care for her. But she was their flesh and blood, not his or the Hospital's, a fact which Bowditch seems to have overlooked in his desire to plan for her a life of usefulness and security.

The story has a moral, in fact two of them. It illustrates and is probably quite typical of the intense personal concern that was felt for the patients at the Massachusetts General Hospital and the McLean Hospital by everyone associated with it from the Trustees and members of the Ladies Visiting Committee to the doctors, nurses, administration and personnel. Trustee Bowditch was really playing the part of a social service worker. The same Yankee sense of duty that had generated such an immediate response to the call of the founders continued to find expression in the daily affairs of the Hospital and does today. Perhaps more than any other institution, the MGH has been the conscience of the community.

But there is a reverse side to the coin. The MGH had been created by one class for the benefit of the community. There was an element of noblesse oblige in the great Trustee's certainty that he knew what was best for an unfortunate little girl, a well-ordered plan for her life in which her family was to play little or no part. For many decades the management of the Hospital remained the prerogative of the privileged classes, for this was the stratum of society from which trustees and doctors alike were drawn. Federalism died slowly in Boston, and the Massachusetts General Hospital, like Harvard College, was a civic possession of the aristocracy.

It must be conceded that if the MGH was born and grew up in the Brahmin tradition, it received the very best that tradition had to offer in terms of financial support, guidance and professional excellence. But by the end of the nineteenth century, both Boston and the MGH were getting too big and complicated to remain the personal charges of any class of citizens. The Hospital was serving more and more patients. An ever growing number was coming for treatment in the clinics; in the decade between 1865 and 1875, for instance, the out-patient load trebled. Advances in medical science were making the care of patients more complex and requiring greater supervision of their convalescence; and they needed increasing assistance in their readjustment to an increasingly kaleidoscopic society. No longer was it possible for those who were managing the Hospital and treating the sick to give effective attention at the same time to the lives and problems of the patients outside of the hospital walls.

THE FIRST MEDICAL SOCIAL SERVICE

In 1905, two years after the opening of its new Out-Patient Building, the Massachusetts General Hospital made one of its greatest contributions to society. In that year, Dr. Richard C. Cabot, the Out-Patient Physician, used private funds to employ two full-time social workers in his department and, with the help of volunteers, started the first medical social service in the world.

Appalled by the enormity of the problems he encountered among the out-patients in his care and the inadequacy of the resources of the MGH and the community to cope with them, Dr. Cabot was struck with the realization that a hospital has a social responsibility for the lives of those affected by sickness which does not start or stop at its doors. He recognized that the time had come for hospitals to enlarge their concept of their place in the community, not merely on a well-meaning, hit-or-miss basis, but as a matter of formal policy. Hospitals should henceforth employ and train experts who would spend all their time helping patients and their families to adjust to the changes which illness and incapacity had brought to their lives.

Dr. Cabot's innovation worked so well that in 1914 his plan was extended to include the bed patients on the wards in addition to the out-patients, and Miss Ida M. Cannon, whose name will always be associated with his in this great social advance, was appointed first Chief of Hospital Social Service. In 1919, after a delay due largely to financial considerations, the Trustees made the Social Service Department an integral part of the hospital organization.

THE PHILLIPS HOUSE FOR PRIVATE PATIENTS

The founders of the Massachusetts General Hospital intended it to be a charitable institution to the extent that most of the patients could not be cared for properly at home or had no home, since many of them were travelers, seafaring men, servants and the like. Certainly the majority were not expected to be able to pay the full cost of their hospitalization, and there were always those who could afford to pay nothing at all.

Doctors donated their services, and the cost of the care of

ward patients was made up out of general hospital funds or by specific funds established by individuals for the support of "free beds." At one time, for example, a subscription of $100 would maintain a bed available to an average of fifteen patients during the year and entitle the donor to nominate the occupants. In the early years, the MGH had to deny admission to some applicants because of the limited number of free beds; but by the middle of the last century it was able to admit all suitable patients regardless of their ability to pay, although they were expected to contribute what they could.

A hundred years ago the conditions on the wards seem to have been reasonably pleasant, and considerable attention — outside of a lack of privacy — appears to have been given the comfort of the patients.

Miss Georgia L. Sturtevant, who later became Matron of the MGH, has left a picture of the conditions that prevailed when she first joined the Hospital as an assistant nurse in 1862. Her initial impression of the life of a nurse was not so favorable:

> I was prepared to see the most shocking sights and sounds, and to be brought face to face with sickness and suffering in every form. But instead of this, I was ushered into a large, bright, airy room, the pretty white-curtained beds, with their strip of bright carpet beside each bed, and in almost every window pretty flowering plants gave the room a most cheerful and homelike appearance. . . .
>
> While the patients, no matter of what nationality, or in what station of life, reposed on dainty, dimity-curtained beds, and used only solid-silver spoons, the nurses, after being on duty for sixteen hours, were shut up in little boxes of rooms between two wards, and sipped their "souchong" — or whatever brand it might have been — from pewter teaspoons, and drank their ice-water, when they were allowed that luxury, from pewter tumblers.

Nevertheless, the hospital was a place to be avoided if one could afford to be sick at home, especially, as we have seen, if surgery was required. But around eighty years ago a change that had gradually been taking place in the complexion of medical care began to be quite obvious. People were getting better treatment in the hospital than was obtainable in their homes, no matter how wealthy they were. The ward patients were reaping the benefits of each new forward step in medicine — and they were coming in quick succession: the aseptic operating room, the x-ray, the laboratory, expert nursing service, the advantages of treatment in an environment of teaching and research.

The most dramatic of these, and the one which more than any other revolutionized public attitudes toward hospitals, was asepsis. Asepsis was the beginning of the end for "hospitalism." With the means at hand to control cross-infection (although currently this has recurred as a problem to some extent), the hospital finally became a safe haven for the sick.

Ironically, the MGH had few accommodations for those who wished to enter as private patients. There were a few private rooms, but they were no match for the growing demand.

As far back as 1863 the Trustees had been aware of this discrepancy and expressed the hope that some rich friend would give the MGH a building for private paying patients "which with every convenience and the privacy of home shall combine that advantage of being attached to a well appointed and well regulated hospital."

But fifty years passed and no friend came forth for the purpose. Meanwhile, the dissatisfaction of many members of the staff over the traditional policy that professional fees charged private patients should be retained by the Hospital had been coming to a head. The Trustees determined to use hospital funds to erect a building for private patients. An important factor behind their decision was the desire to create a private service that would provide the practicing staff with the means of earning all or a substantial part of their living under the same roof where they contributed their services to free patients, taught or carried on research. The Trustees also hoped that admission to the MGH would turn the philanthropy of persons of wealth in its direction.

The new building, with ninety-four beds in comfortable and well-appointed rooms, was opened in 1917 and named the Phillips House in memory of the father and son who were early supporters of the Hospital. Dr. J. Collins Warren, the grandson of the co-founder, was the first patient and was discharged well.

The Phillips House became a reality as part of the rapid growth of the Massachusetts General Hospital during the administration of Dr. Frederic A. Washburn from 1908 to 1934. Dr. Washburn was an imaginative and dynamic leader who conducted the affairs of the Hospital with a spirit of military briskness that made him the natural choice of the Surgeon General to command Base Hospital Number 6, which was organized from the MGH and sent to France in 1917.

In his history of the Hospital from 1900 to 1935, Dr. Washburn referred to himself in the third person as follows:

> Perhaps mention should be made of an amusing incident that occurred about the year 1906. The Assistant Resident Physician (Assistant Director) had recently returned from army service in Porto Rico and the Phillipine Islands. As he observed the House Officers slouching with their hands in their trousers' pockets, he suggested to them from time to time that they try to cure themselves of the habit. As this had no effect, the next lot of white clothes was made with no side pockets in the trousers. This was effectual, but caused a bit of comment and has been a standing joke since.

The pockets, it should be added, have since reappeared.

THE BAKER MEMORIAL FOR PEOPLE OF MODERATE MEANS

With the Phillips House for private patients in the works and the less fortunate provided for in the wards, Dr. Washburn had for some time been concerned about the situation of those in between, the people of moderate means who were too proud to apply or were unqualified for admission to the wards but who couldn't afford hospitalization as private patients. The middle class, he noted in his report of 1914, "must often be ill in their homes, dependent upon physicians who cannot provide the necessary laboratory tests and scientific examinations which are readily available in a general hospital" — a dilemma which at that time was the lot of the wealthy as well.

As luck would have it, Mrs. Mary Rich Richardson bequeathed $1,000,000 to the Hospital in memory of her parents, Richard J. and Ellen Maria Baker. Another $900,000 was raised by public subscription, and in 1930 the 325-bed Baker Memorial Hospital was opened as a unit for patients of moderate means. The Julius Rosenwald Fund provided $150,000 to help meet operating costs for three years, and the Baker Memorial Plan was inaugurated. This plan set up a system of hospital charges which established a moderate scale of professional fees to be included with economy rates so that the patient would have to meet only one all-inclusive bill consistent with his ability to pay.

The Baker Memorial Plan was watched by other hospitals in the country with interest and it was the prototype for similar arrangements where they were feasible. Seven years later the MGH signed its first contract with the Massachusetts Blue Cross, a move which was to bring paid hospitalization within reach of an expanding number of patients.

A hospital as old as the MGH grows in leapfrog fashion. With the opening of the Phillips House and Baker Memorial, the facilities for the care of the wealthy and those of moderate means had jumped overnight from an almost non-existent status to the finest obtainable. Now it was the turn of the ward patients again.

THE GEORGE ROBERT WHITE BUILDING

As we have seen, it did not take the MGH long to outgrow the Bulfinch Building, and the construction of the "Old Brick" in 1854 for isolation patients began a steady proliferation of separate low buildings, each containing a ward. These were connected by passages, and new ones were added on as the patient load increased. This physical separation of the wards was an attempt to avoid the transmittal of infection through the Hospital; they were intended as temporary structures, to be torn down when they got to be "infected." Actually, none were razed until new construction made it necessary. The wards were lettered and also named for noteworthy individuals: A (Warren), B (Jackson), C (Bigelow) and so forth. Being spread out over a considerable area, they were not convenient to central facilities such as operating rooms, laboratories and x-ray, which likewise were in various locations.

In 1930, the year the Baker was opened, the will of Mrs. Harriet J. Bradbury of Boston established the George Robert

White Fund in memory of her brother and provided that a building for the care of the sick should be erected at the Massachusetts General Hospital, its cost not to exceed $2,500,000.

The depression caused delays, but in 1937 the Gay Ward, the Bigelow Surgical Amphitheatre, the Surgical Building and the X-Ray Building were demolished, and workmen began driving pilings down through the filled land which had once been the edge of the Charles River. On October 16, 1939 — Ether Day — the George Robert White Memorial Building was dedicated. It was fourteen stories high, dominating the landscape and proclaiming to the world the location of the MGH. It contained wards, operating rooms, x-ray facilities, laboratories, the emergency ward, administrative offices, kitchens and dining rooms. The White Building pulled things together and became the hub of the Hospital.

MEETING THE NEEDS FOR SPECIALIZED CARE

But the White Building had barely opened before the Massachusetts General Hospital resumed the expansion of its facilities for patients, this time in response to the need for specialized care.

The first move was the establishment through a bequest in 1941 of the Hall-Mercer Hospital for the care and study of psychoneurotic patients, a program which was divided between the MGH and the Pennsylvania Hospital in Philadelphia. The MGH Division was opened in the Bulfinch Building in that year.

The same year the Hospital agreed to erect a new building on its own grounds for the Vincent Memorial Hospital, an institution for the care of women patients. Founded in 1890, it was supported by the Vincent Club of Boston and by endowment and was located in another part of the city. As time went by, the need of the Vincent for the supporting, or ancillary, services of a general hospital could no longer be denied, and the marriage with the MGH was proposed and accepted. Wartime construction restrictions delayed plans. Beds were made available in the White Building, and Dr. Joe Vincent Meigs, Chief Surgeon, was appointed head of the new Gynecology Service. In 1947 the

$1,400,000 Vincent was opened; the upper three floors of the six-story building were dedicated as the Burnham Memorial for Children, made possible by the bequest of Mrs. A. Lawrence Hopkins of a large sum in memory of her god-daughter, Marian Burnham.

The Collis P. Huntington Memorial Hospital moved its program for the treatment and investigation of cancer, including the John Collins Warren Laboratories, to the MGH in 1942, adding its resources to those of the Tumor Clinic, which was the first in the United States when it opened in 1925.

In 1948, Storrow House in Lincoln, gift of the Storrow Estate, was opened as a home in the country for convalescent patients.

Many people assume that the Massachusetts Charitable Eye and Ear Infirmary, next-door neighbor of the MGH and founded in 1827, is a part of the Massachusetts General Hospital. Actually, they are separate corporations, although their close affiliation dates back to 1915 when the director of the MGH was also placed in charge of the Eye and Ear, a dual position that lapsed in 1949. This relationship was further cemented in 1927 when the "Connecting Building" was built between the outpatient departments of the two institutions.

In 1951 the Bay State Rehabilitation Clinic affiliated with the MGH and occupied special quarters that added the advantage of the Hospital's facilities to its extensive program of medical rehabilitation for people disabled by illness.

THE MGH IN WAR AND PEACE

The Massachusetts General Hospital has been called upon to serve the nation and the community during numerous emergencies. The Civil War and World War I have already been mentioned. During the Spanish-American War in 1898 the Hospital pitched tents on the lawn to accommodate many of the 221 men it treated, most of them casualties of typhoid and malaria.

The MGH, along with other hospitals, was scourged by the terrible influenza epidemic of 1918 during the first week of which fifty-seven per cent of all the afflicted patients died.

Eight hundred were admitted, and surgical admissions except emergencies were suspended during the crisis in order to make another 200 beds available.

Soon after the beginning of World War II the Hospital's emergency plan was put to the test on the night of November 28, 1942, when fire swept through the Cocoanut Grove, a Boston night club. Four hundred and ninety-one persons died. One hundred and fourteen were brought to the MGH, thirty-nine remaining alive. Many were saved because adequate supplies of fresh blood and frozen plasma were on hand in the newly organized Blood Bank. New and vastly more effective techniques for the treatment of severe burns that were developed as a result of this catastrophe saved many times more lives during the years of the war that lay ahead.

The following year the MGH was called upon to provide the nation with a military hospital for the second time in a generation. The Sixth General Hospital was organized and served in Africa and Italy under Colonel Thomas R. Goethals. The manpower demands of the Sixth General and of the rest of the armed forces cut the peacetime staff of 312 doctors down to 230, created a serious shortage of nurses and personnel and placed heavy responsibilities on the shoulders of Dr. Nathaniel W. Faxon. Dr. Faxon was Director from 1935 until 1949, when he was succeeded by Dr. Dean A. Clark as General Director.

In 1955 a poliomyelitis epidemic started slowly but built up momentum until it attained the proportions of a full-blown medical crisis. Three hundred and seventy-six adults and fifty-two children were admitted, and entire units of the MGH were temporarily reorganized to cope with the disaster. During the height of the emergency, forty tank respirators were in use simultaneously.

Trends in Nursing

The initial opposition of the Trustees and doctors to the establishment of a school of nursing at the Massachusetts General Hospital ninety years ago — as elsewhere — was probably a reflection of the assumption that the place of every gentlewoman is in the home. Rigid discipline and Calvinistic rules and regulations were imposed. Nurses worked long and arduous hours. They had little to do with the treatment of patients; their job was to keep them clean and comfortable and to perform housekeeping chores.

Before long it began to dawn on the men that, as usual, they had underestimated the determination and the capabilities of the other sex. Dedicated and able nurses refused to accept indefinitely a servant status, compelled the increasing respect of the doctors and patients and made themselves, as time went by, indispensable members of the hospital team. Progress in medicine brought such complexities to the care and treatment of patients that more and more of the responsibilities which had been the prerogative of the doctors were of necessity turned over to the nurses.

Hence, nursing matured as a profession. Student nurses needed education in medical science and years of training to prepare them for critically important responsibilities in specialized areas from the operating room to obstetrics and pediatrics, orthopedics and infectious diseases, administration and teaching.

By the turn of the century the advantage of a college education as a supplement to the course in the MGH School of Nursing was realized, and many students were preparing themselves for a nursing career at Simmons College. By 1937 the times were calling for a new look at the role of the nurse in the MGH. The next year the Trustees adopted the recomendations of Miss Ruth Sleeper (in 1946 to be appointed the Director of the Nursing Service and School of Nursing) that the hours of duty for students should be reduced and that nursing education should be upgraded to the junior college level.

The MGH began a coordinated program of nursing education leading to a degree from Radcliffe College and a diploma from the Hospital; it also participated in the postgraduate education of nurses from Boston University.

The nurses finally were given comfortable and modern quarters in 1953 when Bartlett Hall, a beautiful residence named after the Rev. John Bartlett and built with a bequest from his great-granddaughter, Mary Bartlett Noyes, was opened to relieve the pressure from the Thayer Home erected in 1883 and Walcott House in 1913.

CHAPTER 5

And Gladly Would He Learn, And Gladly Teach

I will look upon him who shall have taught me this Art even as one of my parents . . . I will impart this Art by precept, by lecture, and by every mode of teaching, not only to my own sons, but to the sons of him who has taught me, and to disciples bound by covenant and oath, according to the Law of Medicine.

Down through the centuries these words from the Hippocratic Oath have renewed the inspiration of the student to in turn become the teacher, passing the healing art from hand to hand and from generation to generation. Surely this obligation was uppermost in the minds of James Jackson and John Collins Warren when they observed in the circular letter which is the cornerstone of the Massachusetts General Hospital that the students at the Harvard Medical School "find it impossible to learn some of the most important elements of the science of medicine until after they have undertaken for themselves the care of the health and lives of their fellow citizens."

THE HOUSE PUPILS

Doctors are more made than born; indeed, they make themselves in the process of learning by doing. The medical student, fresh from his initiation into the legacy of science, accompanies his teachers through the hospital, observes their treatment of the patients and assists with many of the duties.

49

Upon the completion of his formal medical education, he comes to live in the hospital and by degrees takes increasing responsibility for the care of patients, always under the close supervision of the experienced members of the staff. This is the way the healing art is passed from hand to hand.

Until the Massachusetts General Hospital admitted its first patient in 1821, the students of the Harvard Medical School and its young graduates followed Doctors Jackson and Warren and other faculty members in their rounds through the Boston Almshouse, a catch-all for the unfortunates of the community which was entirely unsuited either for the care of the sick or for teaching. They were known as House Pupils.

In 1830 the Trustees of the MGH appointed a House Physician and a House Surgeon who were required to have studied medicine for at least a year. They lived at the Hospital and were paid $50 a year. Their number was doubled in 1846, and the educational requirements for these positions were raised. Three years later the term of "House Pupil" was revived; apparently the staff thought they were getting too cocky.

It would appear that these were years when the responsibility of participating in medical education was resting somewhat uneasily on the shoulders of the administration. In 1846 the Trustees told Dr. Warren rather curtly in reply to his request for their opinion about the possibility of the Medical School moving into the vicinity that "they cannot perceive any advantage to this institution to arise therefrom"; as a matter of fact, they added, they could see some distinct disadvantages in the prospect.

Probably the Trustees had in mind the behavior of some of the medical students, many of whom were young bloods disinclined to allow the dignified environment in which they found themselves to interfere with the occasional good times their studies permitted. Now and then a high-spirited riot occurred; there were periodic escapades, annoying if harmless; and of course rumor had it that medical students were not above recruiting subjects for their anatomy classes from the local graveyards.

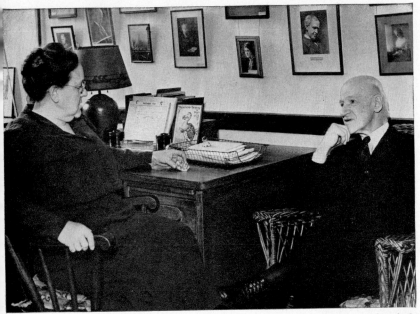

Pioneers in medical social service. Miss Ida M. Cannon and Dr. Richard C. Cabot (1938).

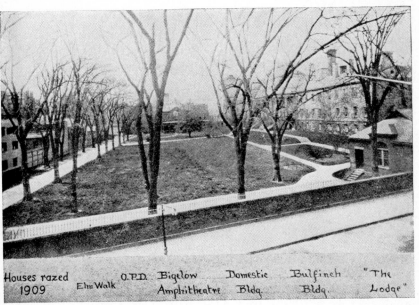

| Houses razed 1909 | Elm Walk | O.P.D. | Bigelow Amphitheatre | Domestic Bldg. | Bulfinch Bldg. | "The Lodge" |

The "Yard" sixty years ago. The George Robert White Building stands on the site of the Bigelow Operating Amphitheatre.

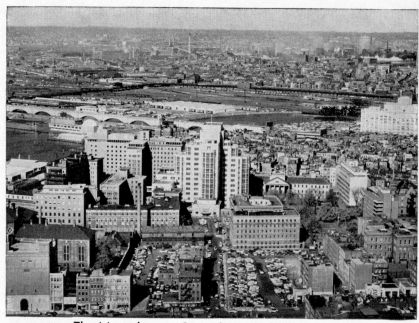

The Massachusetts General Hospital today . . . .

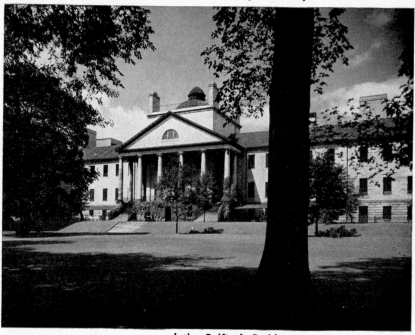

. . . . and the Bulfinch Building

But in spite of the Trustees' lack of enthusiasm, the Harvard Medical School in 1847 moved to a new building on North Grove Street adjacent to the Hospital. It was its third move in sixty-five years, first from the Harvard Yard in Cambridge to a point near Washington and Franklin Streets in downtown Boston in 1810, then in 1816 to a location on Mason Street, finally to the site by the Hospital where it was to remain until 1883.*

By 1858 internal frictions which had been brewing for years came to a head. The House Pupils "revolted" and dispatched a letter to the Trustees, complaining about discipline, the administration, lack of definition of duties of the various staff members and the intervention of the Trustees' Visiting Committee in hospital affairs. The significant result of the uprising was the decision of the Trustees — over the objections of the staff — to appoint a doctor as administrative head of the Hospital for the first time. Dr. Benjamin S. Shaw was named to the position with the title of Resident Physician, and the old post of Superintendent was abolished

As time passed the number of House Pupils was steadily increased, educational requirements were raised and responsibilities were divided among them as needs for specialized training arose. During its first half century the MGH maintained only its general medical and surgical services, a sign of the opposition of the majority of the medical profession to any formal specialization in medicine. But the burgeoning of medical science toward the end of the last century inevitably brought specialization. These changes caused the earlier apprentice type of graduate medical education to give way to the residency system; this advanced the House Pupils through the ranks of general training in medicine or surgery into the particular

*Barely two years after the move to North Grove Street the School was the scene of one of the most electrifying murders in the annals of American crime. Dr. John W. Webster, Erving Professor of Chemistry at the Medical School, having lived beyond his means and being pressed by Dr. George Parkman of the Visiting Staff of the Hospital for payment of a debt, killed his creditor in the Chemical Laboratory during a rage, chopped up the body in a panic and burned it. The murder occurred on November 23, 1849. Dr. Webster was hanged the following year after a sensational trial.

channels of their chosen specialities according to grades of responsibility and the degree to which each specialty required a longer term of hospital service in fulfillment of its demands for competence and experience.

By 1913 a "House Physician" and a "House Surgeon" had been designated to oversee the House Pupils. In 1922 their titles were changed to "resident," the term House Pupil was abandoned for house officer, or intern, and the Resident Physician — in order to avoid further confusion — was thenceforth called Director.

PRESIDENT ELIOT'S REFORM

Much of the incentive behind the continuous upgrading of the house staff of the Massachusetts General Hospital was the result of another "revolution" — this one at Harvard — which brought about improvements in the curriculum at the Medical School and raised the qualifications of its graduates.

It all started when Charles W. Eliot became President of Harvard University in 1869. President Eliot had been unfavorably impressed with instruction at the Medical School during his days of teaching chemistry there, and as part of his general reform of the University's curriculum he went to work on the School with a will. Over the opposition of the old guard on the faculty and with the support of Doctors James C. White, J. Collins Warren and Henry P. Bowditch, President Eliot succeeded in 1870-71 in breaking the Medical School away from the old proprietary system of lectures confined to the winter term and established a three-year graded course of expanded studies patterned after the progressive features of the best in contemporary European medical education.

The Eliot reform breathed new life into the Harvard Medical School; it was forced to find new and larger quarters and in 1883, after thirty-six years on North Grove Street directly opposite the MGH, moved to a location on Boylston Street. This building was soon outgrown, and twenty-five years later the School moved again to its present impressive group of marble buildings on Longwood Avenue. The physical removal of the

Medical School from the neighborhood of the Massachusetts General Hospital coincided with the realization that it would have to look to other institutions in addition to the MGH for clinical facilities; locations more central to the growing number of hospitals in Boston were advantageous for this purpose without impairing the close relationship between Harvard and the MGH.

THE CPC: A NEW TEACHING METHOD

A superb example of the subtle way an environment of teaching and investigation can catalyze new ideas and nurture them into major innovations began in 1895 when Dr. Richard C. Cabot, who was later to devise medical social service, started to use printed case histories of patients as private quiz exercises for his students. After about five years he brought this teaching method to the Harvard Medical School. In 1910, in cooperation with Dr. J. Homer Wright, the Hospital's Pathologist, Dr. Cabot initiated weekly clinical pathological conferences.

The clinical pathological conference, or CPC, was a significant contribution to medical education. Here is how it works: the history of a patient with a challenging problem whose case has gone to autopsy or operation is presented before a group of doctors or medical students; it is discussed by experts who, on the basis of the facts presented, offer their diagnosis; this is compared with the diagnosis actually made by the doctors who attended the patient; then the pathologist presents and explains his findings (these have been withheld from the discussants and the audience) based on the actual illness as confirmed by autopsy or operation. It is a game of highly educated guessing in which only the pathologist knows the answer beforehand. It offers students an invaluable opportunity to study the mental processes that are involved in making a diagnosis and at the same time sharpens and refreshes the diagnostic instinct of the experienced doctor who attends the CPC or reads an account of it and tests himself.

The invention of Doctors Cabot and Wright caught on immediately and was incorporated into the clinical curriculum of the Medical School. Dr. Cabot next published collections in book form; then he found himself mailing accounts of CPC's to readers who requested them from all over the world. Finally, they were published every week as the "Case Records of the Massachusetts General Hospital" in the *Boston Medical and Surgical Journal,* later to become the *New England Journal of Medicine,* and they have carried the name of the MGH to the remotest corners of the globe. Recently a traveling staff member reported that he had found the "Case Records" being studied in the middle of the Saudi-Arabian desert, and doctors in several countries have formed clubs for the purpose of discussing these exercises after the arrival of the weekly *Journal.*

How to Support Teaching and Research in a Hospital?

In recent years the Massachusetts General Hospital has helped to provide many doctors on the faculty of the Harvard Medical School with a means of earning part of the income from the practice of medicine that enables them to donate varying amounts of their time to teaching. The organization of the staff has remained flexible so that the Hospital could adapt itself to changing conditions and maintain its ability to attract and keep men and women having a strong interest in teaching and research in addition to the care of patients.

The two medical services of the Hospital were united in 1921 under Dr. David L. Edsall as Chief. When he resigned to become the first full-time Dean of Harvard Medical School, he was succeeded in this position in 1923 by Dr. James Howard Means. Upon his retirement in 1951 Dr. Means was succeeded by Dr. Walter Bauer. A similar union of the surgical services came in 1948 under Dr. Edward D. Churchill.

The financial support of the teacher in a hospital that is attempting to hold down rising costs of medical care presented numerous difficulties during the inflationary postwar period. By 1949 the MGH and Harvard had undertaken a series of discussions from which emerged a new policy defining their joint responsibility for the support of the members of the teaching staff at the Hospital according to their degree of participation in this activity.

During the decade of the nineteen fifties the MGH and Harvard concentrated on working out ways of expanding their program of teaching and research and of assigning emphasis and costs in such a manner that each would bear a realistic share of the burden, placing as little of it as possible on the patient.

Government assistance to hospitals and support of medical research was a reality, and indeed the modern university medical center could not carry on its program without this aid. The MGH had received large sums of money under the Hill-Burton Act for construction, and more than half of its research funds was comprised of grants from the National Institutes of Health and other Federal agencies.

But it was believed as a matter of policy that the viability of the MGH and every other medical center as free institutions depended upon the balancing of government support by the continued voluntary assistance of society.

A Productive Partnership

Harvard was fortunate that the MGH was conceived as a teaching hospital and that its destinies were guided by men who sensed the advantages to their community of this relationship and were careful to perpetuate it.

By the same token, the MGH owes its existence to Harvard's need and many of its achievements to the excellence of the Medical School's teachers and graduates. The quality of the service it has rendered the community has been influenced historically by the superlative standards of medicine which the School has always set for itself and insisted upon in the hospitals with which it is affiliated.

Both the MGH and Harvard have reason to be thankful that the Hospital has remained an independent institution, free from the supervision of the Medical School, while the University has escaped the burden of operating a hospital for the incidental benefit of its medical students. The two have been at liberty to fulfill the functions that were defined for each, working together wherever these purposes coincided.

The rationale behind this relationship was supplied by James Jackson and John Collins Warren and has prevailed for a century and a half. The partnership has been productive in three respects: it has given patients care of the highest quality; in the Hippocratic tradition it has helped to renew continuously the life blood of medicine in Boston, in America and throughout the world; and it has created an atmosphere that excites keen minds to explore the dark continents of disease.

THE END